D0512795

What you really need to know about

IRRITABLE
BOWEL
SYNDROME

Dr. Robert Buckman
with Nigel Howard
Introduced by John Cleese

MARSHALL PUBLISHING

A Marshall Edition
Conceived by Marshall Editions
The Orangery
161 New Bond Street
London W1Y 9PA

First published in the UK in 2000 by
Marshall Publishing Ltd
Copyright © 2000 Marshall Editions Developments Ltd

ISBN: 1 84028 345 9

Originated in Italy by Articolor
Printed and bound in Italy by New Interlitho

Managing Editor Theresa Reynolds
Indexer Susan Bosanko
Art Editor Siân Keogh
Illustrator Martin Laurie
Photographer Martin Norris
Managing Editor Anne Yelland
Managing Art Editor Helen Spencer
Editorial Director Ellen Dupont
Art Director Dave Goodman
Editorial Coordinator Ros Highstead
Production Nikki Ingram, Anna Pauletti

Cover photography: front Superstock; back Dick Luria/ Telegraph Colour Library

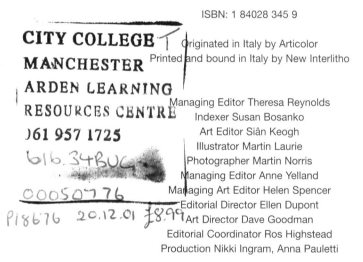
The consultant for this book, Dr. Paul Maxwell, BSc, MBBS, MRCP, is a specialist registrar
in Gastroenterology in the South Thames Region and a clinical research fellow
at St. Georges Hospital Medical School. Dr. Maxwell specializes in research into
the epidemiology and pathophysiology of IBS.

Contents

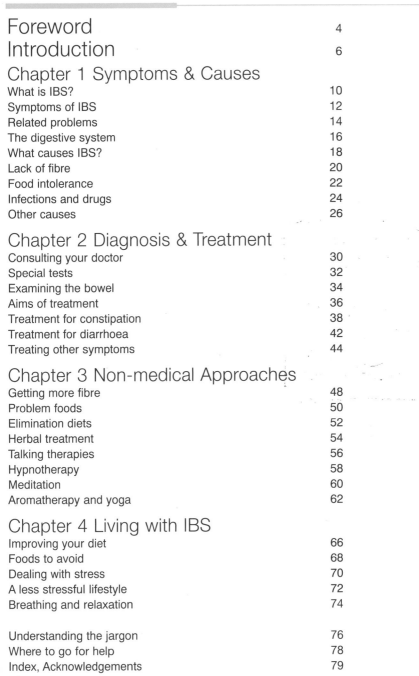

Foreword

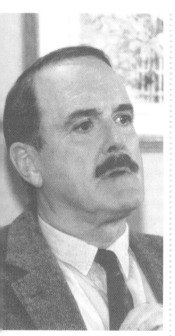

Most of you know me best as someone who makes people laugh.

But for 30 years I have also been involved with communicating information. And one particular area in which communication often breaks down is the doctor/patient relationship. We have all come across doctors who fail to communicate clearly, using complex medical terms when a simple explanation would do, and dismiss us with a "come back in a month if you still feel unwell". Fortunately, I met Dr Robert Buckman.

Rob is one of North America's leading experts on cancer, but far more importantly he is a doctor who believes that hiding behind medical jargon is unhelpful and unprofessional. He wants his patients to understand what is wrong with them, and spends many hours with them—and their families and close friends—making sure they understand everything. Together we created a series of videos, with the jargon-free title *Videos for Patients*. Their success has prompted us to write books that explore medical conditions in the same clear, simple terms.

This book is one of a series that will tell you all you need to know about your condition. It assumes nothing. If you have a helpful, honest, communicative doctor, you will find here the extra information that he or she simply may not have time to tell you. If you are less fortunate, this book will help to give you a much clearer picture of your situation.

More importantly—and this was a major factor in the success of the videos—you can access the information here again and again. Turn back, read over, until you really know what your doctor's diagnosis means.

In addition, because in the middle of a consultation, you may not think of everything you would like to ask your doctor, you can also use the book to help you formulate the questions you would like to discuss with him or her.

John Cleese

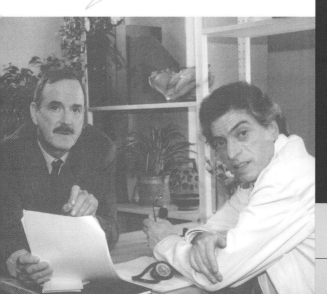

Introduction

As the title says, this book aims to tell you what you really need to know about an extremely common health problem, irritable bowel syndrome or IBS for short. It does not attempt to cram every last theory, piece of research or diet fad between its covers. Instead, it cuts through the mass of confusing information that surrounds IBS to give you the basic facts about this distressing and often misunderstood condition.

How the book works

The book describes the symptoms of IBS, outlines what little is known about its causes and explains how your doctor will go about making a diagnosis. It then goes on to show how, once you have been diagnosed as having IBS, you can take action to overcome the problem by making changes in your lifestyle.

Taking action

A few people with IBS are able to identify a particular trigger for their symptoms, such as a food to which they are sensitive, and avoid it. However, for most sufferers from IBS life is not that simple because the cause of their symptoms cannot be determined.

If you belong to this majority, don't despair. It may take longer but, as this book shows, there are still plenty of approaches which can help you to reduce your symptoms in the long term, though you may not be able to banish them altogether.

If your symptoms are particularly troublesome, medical treatment from your doctor, explained in Chapter Two, will help, albeit as a short-term measure. Once your symptoms have been eased, you can start looking for a way to reduce their frequency and severity.

Coping with the condition

Irritable bowel syndrome is what is known as a paroxysmal condition, which is a medical way of saying that it comes and goes, with the symptoms entirely absent at some times, then becoming very severe. The symptoms and severity of IBS vary considerably from person to person but for most individuals the condition follows a pattern of rumbling along, causing the occasional problem, then flaring up for a while before subsiding again.

Obviously the ideal solution is to find out what is triggering your symptoms. Some of the approaches explained in Chapter Three can help you do this. You can take steps to prevent your symptoms from flaring up again. Chapter Four looks at basic diet and lifestyle changes which can help you achieve this.

THE IBS NETWORK

Reliable, up-to-date information on IBS can be hard to come by, and many sufferers find the services provided by the IBS Network of great help. The Network is a self-help organization for people with irritable bowel syndrome. It produces fact sheets and a quarterly journal, *Gut Reaction*, covering a wide variety of topics relating to IBS. It operates befriender and penfriend schemes, runs therapeutic group programmes and co-ordinates local self-help groups. Members also have the opportunity to participate in medical research and join a media list or reviewing scheme. You can find contact details for the IBS Network on page 78.

Chapter

SYMPTOMS & CAUSES

What is IBS?

Irritable bowel syndrome, or IBS for short, is an extremely common digestive disorder. Its symptoms can include abdominal pain, bloating, constipation and diarrhoea. The symptoms can be mild, or they can be serious enough to interfere with everyday life.

How serious is IBS?

IBS may be uncomfortable and unpleasant but it is not life-threatening. However, it does share some symptoms with other, more serious disorders of the bowel such as ulcerative colitis (inflammation and ulceration of the large intestine) or Crohn's disease (inflammation of the lower part of the small intestine). It is therefore important to have your condition diagnosed by a doctor to exclude the possibility that you have one of these conditions.

How common is IBS?

If you have IBS you are not alone. In the developed countries of the world between 13 and 22 percent of the population have symptoms of IBS at some time or another, and one in 10 people are affected seriously enough to seek medical help. Irritable bowel syndrome is the most common reason for people to be referred by their GP to specialist gastroenterology clinics. In Britain, for example, more than half of the patients attending such clinics have IBS.

Who suffers from IBS?

IBS affects people of all ages; symptoms usually first appear between the ages of 15 and 40. In the UK, more women than men are affected, and women are also more likely to consult their GP about symptoms. (This is not universal; in India, more men than women are affected.)

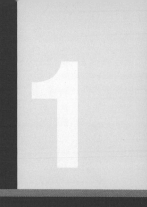

SOME COMMON MISCONCEPTIONS

MYTH	REALITY
"IBS IS HEREDITARY."	Other members of the family may have similar symptoms but you do not have an increased risk of suffering from IBS just because your parents did.
"YOU CAN CATCH IBS FROM A BACTERIA OR VIRUS."	It is not caused by an infection with a bacteria or virus, although it can sometimes be triggered by a bout of "holiday tummy" or gastroenteritis.
"ONCE YOU GET IBS, YOUR CONDITION WILL DETERIORATE OVER TIME."	IBS is not a progressive disorder; in other words it does not get worse as time goes by. Instead, it is there, grumbling away in the background, occasionally flaring up and then subsiding.
"IBS IS NOT A REAL ILLNESS—IT'S ALL IN THE MIND."	Like many health problems, IBS can be made worse by stress and anxiety but its symptoms result from a physical disorder.

YOU REALLY NEED TO KNOW

◆ IBS is a common digestive disorder affecting mainly young and middle-aged adults, though it can occur at any age.

◆ Symptoms may be mild, and not all sufferers seek their doctor's help.

◆ IBS is not life-threatening, infectious, progressive or all in the mind.

What is IBS?

Symptoms of IBS

FACTS

✓ Many people suffer some of the symptoms of IBS from time to time, but don't have the syndrome.

✗ IBS sufferers experience symptoms over a long period of time — occasional bouts of constipation, diarrhoea or abdominal pain don't amount to IBS.

Irritable bowel syndrome is not a disease in the true sense of the word. It is a condition or disorder. "Syndrome" is the medical term for a group of symptoms which often occur together and are associated with a single disorder.

The symptoms of IBS vary between individuals and from time to time. Some people experience an occasional abdominal pain and need to rush to the toilet first thing in the morning to empty their bowels, while others suffer the full range of symptoms. All those with IBS will experience some or all of the symptoms discussed here.

Abdominal pain or discomfort

This can be experienced either as a continuous dull ache or in the form of cramps, both of which come and go in waves. Pain and discomfort can occur anywhere in the

WHAT DOES IT MEAN?

CONSTIPATION

Constipation is usually defined as having a bowel motion less than twice a week or straining to pass stools (faeces) more than 25 per cent of the time.

DIARRHOEA

Diarrhoea is defined as a loose consistency of stool with increased frequency of bowel motions lasting longer than two weeks.

SYNDROME

A collection of symptoms that often occur together and are associated with a single disorder.

abdominal area, although this tends to be worse low down on the left-hand side. The pain generally comes on after eating and is worse during bouts of constipation. It is frequently relieved by opening the bowels or by passing wind.

Bloating

IBS sufferers often experience feelings of abdominal bloating, so that clothes feel tight and uncomfortable. The bloating sensation may be accompanied by rumbling noises and flatulence (wind). It is often triggered by eating, and may get worse over the course of a day.

Constipation and diarrhoea

Of the two, constipation is more common in IBS sufferers, though sometimes constipation and diarrhoea alternate in the same individual. These symptoms are often accompanied by pain. In some people diarrhoea comes on after a meal or when they wake up in the morning, and the need to empty the bowels may be so urgent that they cannot reach the toilet in time.

Other changes in the stools

Stools can become small, hard and pellet-like and can be covered in mucus—the mucus glands in the bowel walls become overstimulated by prolonged contact with slow-moving stools. It is not uncommon to just pass mucus.

A feeling of incomplete emptying

After going to the toilet, sufferers from IBS may still feel they need to empty their bowels. This can lead to ineffective straining to pass further stools and may trigger a sharp, cramping pain deep in the rectum (back passage).

YOU REALLY NEED TO KNOW

◆ IBS is not a disease, it is a condition or disorder.

◆ Symptoms vary from person to person and from time to time.

◆ Sufferers from IBS may experience only some of the symptoms mentioned.

Related problems

Sometimes IBS symptoms can lead to further problems. Constantly straining to pass stools because of constipation, for example, can lead to haemorrhoids (piles). IBS sufferers often experience other disorders which, although not directly caused by their bowel problems, are thought to be related to the syndrome.

Anal fissure

Very large hard stools can tear the anal canal lining as they pass through, especially if they are passed quickly. There is usually some pain as the stool is passed, a little

HAEMORRHOIDS (PILES)

Straining to pass stools due to constipation may damage the veins in and around the anus; the valves give way and the veins become dilated (this is exactly what happens with varicose veins in the legs). A soft lump forms which may feel uncomfortable, though is rarely painful. Piles may develop inside the anus or on its outer edge. They may be damaged and bleed when stools pass over them. If the blood trapped in an external pile clots, the pile may become extremely painful. A doctor can anaesthetize the area and remove the clot.

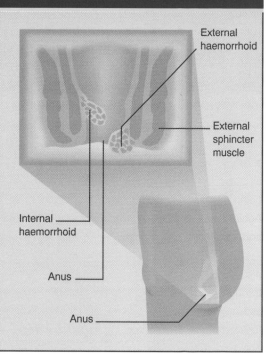

External haemorrhoid

External sphincter muscle

Internal haemorrhoid

Anus

Anus

bleeding, and more pain on passing stools subsequently. The pain can make the sufferer put off passing stools, which makes constipation worse.

The tear may heal of its own accord within a few days; if not, a doctor can prescribe a local anaesthetic cream to numb the area until it does. A chronic fissue may require treatment under general anaesthetic.

Nausea and belching

Although not typical of IBS, nausea is a problem for some sufferers. It may be caused by wind travelling upward from the bowels and causing spasm in the small intestine. Strictly speaking, however, nausea and belching are not symptoms of IBS; they may be symptoms of anxiety and depression, which are more common in IBS sufferers than in non-sufferers.

Other symptoms

IBS sufferers commonly experience non-intestinal symptoms. The range is wide: tiredness and lethargy, urinary frequency and urgency, recurrent back and loin pain, painful sexual intercourse, chest pain and palpitations, shortness of breath, wheezing and hyperventilation have all been reported. This has led in the past to sufferers being dismissed as hypochondriacs, or to misdiagnosis. Again, some of these symptoms may be due to anxiety and depression.

Research has confirmed, however, that IBS sufferers are more likely to develop some of these symptoms throughout life. They are also more likely to develop asthma. One study found that 22.4 percent of IBS sufferers had over-sensitive lung airways, compared with only 12.2 percent in non-sufferers.

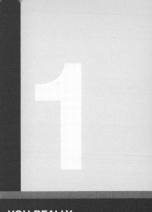

YOU REALLY NEED TO KNOW

◆ Anal bleeding is not in itself a symptom of IBS, but may be caused by piles or an anal fissure arising from constipation.

◆ Continuous bleeding from the anus is never a symptom of IBS and should be investigated by a doctor as it can be a symptom of a more serious disorder.

◆ Seemingly unrelated symptoms, from sexual difficulties to shortness of breath, are often associated with IBS symptoms.

Related problems

The digestive system

A brief look at the digestive system and at the workings of the bowel in particular will help explain how the symptoms of IBS occur.

The digestive tract

The bowel forms part of the digestive tract, a long, muscular tube which runs from the mouth to the anus and forms the body's system for taking in and breaking down food, absorbing the nutrients it provides and disposing of the leftover waste. The internal walls of the tract are protected from general wear and tear by a coating of

SECTIONS OF THE DIGESTIVE TRACT

The digestive tract is divided into several sections, each of which has a specialized function. These are, from top to bottom, the oesophagus, the stomach, the small intestine (which itself comprises three sections: the duodenum, the jejunum and the ileum), the large intestine, (caecum, colon and the rectum). Together these make up the digestive system. The liver, gall bladder and pancreas are also important in the process of digestion, as they supply the chemicals which help the bowel break down food.

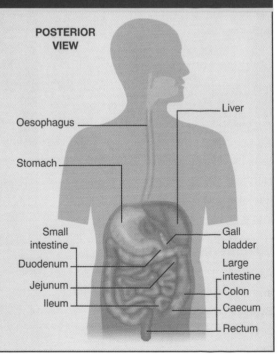

POSTERIOR VIEW

Oesophagus
Stomach
Small intestine
Duodenum
Jejunum
Ileum
Liver
Gall bladder
Large intestine
Colon
Caecum
Rectum

slippery mucus which also helps food slide along smoothly. The job of the digestive tract is to propel the food we eat from mouth to anus, allowing the body to absorb and digest nutrients along the way.

How food is digested

As we chew food it becomes mixed with saliva, allowing it to be swallowed. The chewed food enters the throat and is pushed down through the oesophagus by rhythmic contractions until it reaches the stomach. There it is broken down by acidic gastric juices over a period of several hours into proteins, starches, fats and sugars; complex fats and sugars begin to be broken down here.

When the food is reduced to a semi-liquid state, contractions of the stomach's muscular walls push it down into the small intestine. Here what remains of our meal is further digested, this time by alkaline juices, chemicals from the liver, gall bladder and pancreas and colonies of friendly bacteria.

Absorption of nutrients

By the time it reaches the end of the small intestine, the food has been reduced to a few simple chemicals. Nutrients are absorbed into the body through the walls of the small intestine and the leftover slurry is pushed on into the large intestine.

Waste disposal

As the leftovers pass through the large intestine, water and salts are absorbed into the body through its walls. By the time the waste matter arrives in the rectum, it has become a soft, solid material ready to be expelled during the next bowel motion.

What causes IBS?

The symptoms of IBS are caused by changes in the way the bowel works, not by a specific disease. In IBS the bowel is found to be completely normal on examination but behaves abnormally from time to time. For this reason, doctors classify IBS as a "functional disorder" to distinguish it from "organic disorders" such as inflammatory bowel disease.

Triggers

Despite years of research, it is still unclear why the bowel should misbehave in these ways in people with IBS. It may well be that IBS is triggered by different things in different people. Known triggers include lack of dietary fibre, food intolerance, infections, antibiotics and other

DIGESTION IN IBS SUFFERERS

Any disruption to the regular contractions that propel digested food through the large intestine can result in the symptoms of IBS. The nature of the disruption determines which of the possible symptoms will be experienced.

SYMPTOM	CAUSE
DIARRHOEA	Contents of large intestine pushed through too quickly, so there is not enough time for water to be removed.
CONSTIPATION	Contents of large intestine pushed through too slowly, so too much water is extracted.
ABDOMINAL PAIN	Walls of intestine suddenly contract in spasms.

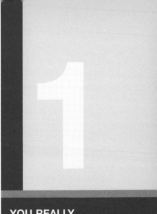

A NERVE DISORDER

IBS is a disorder in the way in which the nerves that link the brain and bowel work; this is the key to understanding the condition. The gut becomes hypersensitive, behaving exactly as in "normal" people, but with less provocation. For example, many people suffer diarrhoea because of the adrenaline release associated with a job interview; in an IBS sufferer, even the small amount of adrenaline associated with a shopping trip could cause the same result. The sensations sufferers receive from their bowel may be more intense than those experienced by non-sufferers. Research shows that some individuals with IBS feel discomfort and pain when their rectums are less full of stool than would cause the same symptoms in a non-sufferer. Unfortunately, we still do not know for sure what causes this hypersensitivity.

drugs, stress, menstruation and smoking. Because IBS is a disorder of the digestive system, many people believe that the role of food is crucial.

A real illness

Until recently, the fact that IBS sufferers appeared physically healthy led the medical profession to believe that their symptoms were due to psychological problems. Doctors believed that the personality of sufferers led them to misinterpret normal fluctuations in bowel function as symptoms of disease. This view is becoming less common. Most experts now believe that the symptoms of IBS result from a real physical malfunction.

Lack of fibre

Fibre is the part of our food that we cannot digest. Fruits and vegetables and grains such as wheat, rye, rice and millet are all rich in fibre. Fibre is an important part of our diet because it passes through the digestive system into the large intestine where it makes the stools bulkier. This speeds their passage through the intestine and into the rectum and makes them easier to pass as stools.

Lack of fibre means that the stools are smaller and, as a result, the walls of the large intestine have to contract more tightly to propel them along. This slows down the system and results in constipation.

Why we lack fibre

The rise in the popularity of processed and "convenience" foods in recent decades has resulted in a steady fall in the amount of fibre in our diets. Many experts blame this decrease in dietary fibre for the increase in the so-called "Western" diseases. These include bowel cancer, gallstones, haemorrhoids (piles), constipation and especially diverticulosis—a very common condition in which the bowel's mucous lining breaks through the outer muscle layers. causing outpouchings of the bowel wall, and leading to symptoms similar to those of IBS.

The role of fibre in treatment

Today fibre supplements, known as bulking agents, are an established part of IBS treatment. Certainly many people with IBS find that increasing their intake of dietary fibre helps their symptoms. However, others find too much fibre or the wrong type can make things worse. Many people find they are unable to tolerate gluten, a protein in wheat bran, the most common form of fibre in the Western diet (see p.23).

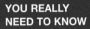

THE REDISCOVERY OF FIBRE

Scientific interest in the role of fibre in bowel problems was sparked by research carried out in Africa in the early 1970s. Bowel problems were known to be far less common among Africans living in rural areas who ate a diet naturally rich in fibre and low in refined and processed foods than they were in the industrial societies of the Western world. The researchers found that, compared to typical Americans or Europeans, the rural Africans had a faster digestive process and heavier stools.

Scientists investigating the effects of bran and other forms of dietary fibre then found that it reduced constipation, and fibre became the watchword for those who wished to eat a healthy diet.

The current recommended fibre intake for adults is 18 grams a day. This amount can be provided by two slices of wholemeal bread, a 110 gram portion of baked beans, and a large (170 grams) apple, orange or banana.

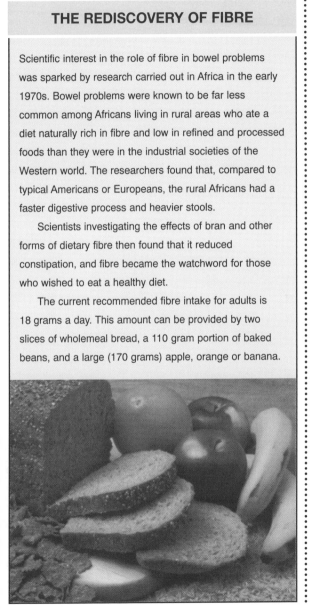

YOU REALLY NEED TO KNOW

◆ An adequate intake of fibre can help with the symptoms of IBS.

◆ Most people eat only two-thirds of the recommended daily intake of 18 g fibre a day.

◆ Processed and convenience foods tend to be low in fibre.

Lack of fibre

Food intolerance

Some sufferers from IBS find that certain foods trigger their symptoms.

Not all sensitivities to food are caused by an allergic reaction.

When people find that a specific type of food disagrees with them they often say they are allergic to it. People with IBS frequently say their symptoms are triggered or at least made worse by certain foods and drinks.

This is possible but an allergy is not to blame. An allergy is a physical reaction which results when the body's immune system attacks a foreign substance. Asthma and eczema are common conditions involving allergic reactions. To date, researchers have not been able to find such a reaction with IBS. The problem is therefore a food intolerance rather than an allergy.

How foods may trigger symptoms

There are many theories about how certain foods could cause the symptoms of IBS in some people in the absence of an allergic reaction. One theory suggests that

PROBLEM FOODS AND DRINKS

Diarrhoea is one of the symptoms that can be caused by intolerance to the following foods and drinks:

- caffeine-containing drinks such as coffee, tea and colas

- chocolate

- dairy products: milk, soft cheese, yoghurt, ice cream

- fruit juices and soft fruit drinks

- sugar-free gum and mints containing sorbitol or mannitol

- dates and figs

- nuts

the symptoms of IBS may be a reaction to potentially toxic substances found in everyday food, such as the flavour-enhancer monosodium glutamate, caffeine, additives such as tartrazine, and the chemicals tyramine and histamine, both found in cheese.

Chemicals known as enzymes are produced by the digestive system to break down these substances and render them harmless. Some researchers believe that people with IBS produce fewer of such enzymes, leaving them vulnerable to the toxic effects of these substances.

The role of food intolerance in IBS remains contro-versial. In general, gut-stimulating foods will have a greater effect on IBS sufferers than on non-sufferers, with caffeine the worst offender. Cutting out such foods may improve symptoms for many people (see pp.50–53).

Lactose intolerance

Those affected by lactose intolerance, which is caused by an enzyme deficiency, do not produce enough of the enzyme lactase which is needed to digest lactose, a sugar found in milk. Lactose intolerance results in IBS-like symptoms of diarrhoea, stomach pain, bloating and wind.

Coeliac disease

People with coeliac disease cannot tolerate gluten, a protein found in cereals such as wheat, barley, rye and oats. This interferes with the proper digestion of food, leading to malnourishment. Symptoms usually improve quickly on a gluten-free diet.

Coeliac disease may not be identified until adulthood and affects up to 2 percent of the population. Some of its symptoms are similar to those of IBS, but new tests have made it much easier to confirm the diagnosis.

YOU REALLY NEED TO KNOW

◆ Certain common foods may cause or worsen symptoms of IBS.

◆ The reaction to the problem food is not an allergy, as it does not involve the immune system.

◆ Food intolerances such as lactose intolerance and coeliac disease can cause IBS-like symptoms, so a proper diagnosis is essential.

Infections and drugs

DOs AND DON'Ts

Do consult your doctor if you experience side effects from any medicines.

Don't stop taking antibiotics because of side effects, or the infection they are meant to treat could recur. If side effects are worrying you, see your doctor.

The symptoms of IBS can sometimes be caused by an illness affecting the bowels, the treatment given to cure it, or drugs given for other conditions.

Infections

Many cases of IBS seem to start after a bout of gastroenteritis ("holiday tummy"), which is usually caused by a bacterial infection. The invading bacteria can upset the balance of micro-organisms in the bowel.

Antibiotics

Some people develop symptoms of IBS after taking a course of antibiotics. Antibiotics kill disease-causing bacteria. But they can also destroy micro-organisms that

COMMON DRUGS WHICH CAN AFFECT BOWEL FUNCTION

DRUG/INGREDIENT	PRODUCT	SYMPTOM/SIDE EFFECT
MAGNESIUM	Some antacids	Diarrhoea
CODEINE	Some painkillers and cough medicines	Constipation
ASPIRIN, IBUPROFEN	Painkillers with an anti-inflammatory action	Diarrhoea, abdominal pain
CAFFEINE	Some headache and hangover remedies	Diarrhoea
IMIPRAMINE, NORTRIPTYLINE ETC.	Tricyclic antidepressants	Constipation

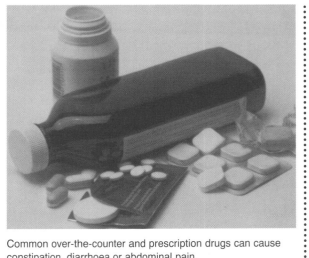

Common over-the-counter and prescription drugs can cause constipation, diarrhoea or abdominal pain.

live in the digestive system, upsetting the delicate bacterial balance that aids the digestion of food. There is no definitive scientific evidence as yet that antibiotics cause IBS, and the connection has still to be proved.

Other drugs

Various other drugs can affect the way in which the bowel works. If you develop IBS symptoms while taking any drug, whether prescribed by your doctor or bought over the counter in a pharmacy, read the information on side effects in the accompanying leaflet or on the package to see whether it could be causing the problem. If in doubt, consult your doctor or pharmacist. Never discontinue prescribed drugs without your doctor's advice.

The effects of drugs are not always clear-cut. Tricyclic antidepressants, which can cause constipation in some people, can also be an excellent treatment for some IBS sufferers (see p.44).

YOU REALLY NEED TO KNOW

◆ Certain infections and drugs affect the bowel and may cause symptoms of IBS.

◆ You should consult your doctor if you experience any side effects as a result of taking prescribed or over-the-counter drugs.

Other causes

Other factors besides diet, illness and drugs can cause or worsen the symptoms of IBS. These include stress, menstruation and smoking cigarettes.

Stress

It is unlikely that stress by itself causes IBS, but many sufferers say that their symptoms are aggravated during periods of anxiety and tension. This is hardly surprising, as we know that stress can have a powerful effect on the functioning of the bowels.

When we experience a stressful event, powerful chemicals are produced in the body—the so-called "fight or flight" hormones, of which adrenaline is the best known. These ready the body for action. They prompt rapid breathing to fill the blood with oxygen and increase the heart rate and blood pressure in order to speed the freshly oxygenated blood to the muscles.

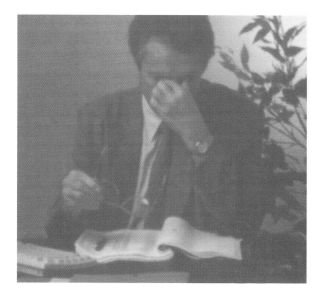

Most people will suffer a bout of diarrhoea when faced with a stressful work situation. Learning a relaxation technique can help avoid aggravating your IBS symptoms (see pp.72–75).

The "fight or flight" hormones also have a direct effect on the digestive system, making the bowel contract more rapidly. This can result in a feeling of churning or "butterflies" in the stomach and, in especially alarming circumstances, in sudden diarrhoea.

Many people with IBS find that self-help to reduce their stress levels eases or even banishes their symptoms.

Female sex hormones

Many women with IBS find that their symptoms are worse during their periods. The reason is unclear, although it is thought to be an effect of the female sex hormones, oestrogen and progesterone, on the digestive system.

Research also suggests that the speed at which the bowel contracts to move food along varies at different stages of the menstrual cycle as the relative levels of these two hormones alter. In the second half of the menstrual cycle (following ovulation), food can take up to twice as long to pass through the gut.

Some researchers have noted a connection between IBS and hysterectomy (surgical removal of the womb); 10 percent of women who have a hysterectomy go on to develop IBS symptoms. However, this may be due to the antibiotics given after the operation to prevent infection rather than the effect of the surgery on hormone levels.

Smoking

Nicotine can interfere with the normal working of the bowel. It has a direct effect on the nerves controlling bowel-wall contractions and can alter their natural pattern. Many people with IBS find that smoking cigarettes or even sitting in a smoky atmosphere makes their symptoms worse.

Other causes

Chapter

2

DIAGNOSIS & TREATMENT

Consulting your doctor

✔ Keep a detailed record of your symptoms for a week or more before consulting your doctor—this will help him or her to make a diagnosis.

✗ Don't hesitate to ask your doctor questions if there's anything you don't understand or are worried about.

When you consult a doctor about your symptoms of IBS, his or her first concern will be to make sure you do not have a more serious bowel disorder. This is because problems such as inflammatory bowel disease and cancer can cause similar symptoms to those of IBS.

What will my doctor need to know?

Your doctor will ask you about your medical history and symptoms, including how long you have been experiencing them and how often, and will give you a thorough physical examination and do some blood tests.

What examinations will be carried out?

If you are under 45 and have not unexpectedly lost weight recently, your doctor will probably keep investigations to a minimum.

The doctor will examine your abdomen with his or her hands. In IBS this normally does not reveal anything unusual apart from a slight tenderness.

The doctor will also carry out a rectal examination using a gloved index finger and a water-based lubricating gel. This can be slightly uncomfortable but is not painful. In IBS the rectum will appear completely normal, so this examination is mainly to rule out other, more serious conditions, including cancer.

A blood sample will be taken and checked for such problems as infections and anaemia.

What is normal bowel function?

In asking about your symptoms, your doctor is trying to establish whether your bowel function is normal. Normal bowel function varies greatly from one person to another and also for any individual at different times. Anything

GUIDELINES FOR DIAGNOSIS

An internationally agreed system, the Rome Criteria, is used to diagnose IBS and distinguish it from other bowel disorders. This states that, in order to make a diagnosis of IBS, there must be at least three months' continuous or recurrent abdominal pain or discomfort which is:

◆ eased by bowel movement

◆ and/or associated with a change in frequency of bowel movement

◆ and/or associated with a change in the consistency of stool

plus two or more of the following on at least a quarter of all bowel movements

◆ altered frequency of bowel movement

◆ altered stool form (that is, lumpy/hard or loose/watery)

◆ altered stool passage (straining, urgency or a feeling of incomplete evacuation)

◆ passage of mucus

◆ a feeling of bloating

YOU REALLY NEED TO KNOW

◆ Your doctor will need to rule out the possibility of other bowel conditions before making a diagnosis of IBS.

◆ You may have to have a painless internal examination and a blood test.

◆ A diagnosis of IBS cannot be made unless the symptoms have persisted for at least three months.

from two or three bowel movements a week to two or three a day is considered normal. The form and consistency of the stools is also important; small, separate hard lumps ("rabbit droppings") and mushy or watery stools are both considered abnormal.

Special tests

If you are over 45 and your symptoms have begun recently, the doctor will normally refer you to a specialist for more extensive tests to exclude other disorders. These tests (and the ones on pp.34–35) will be carried out in the gastroenterology out-patients department of your local hospital. They may include an internal examination of your bowel with a special viewing instrument and laboratory tests to check for blood in the stools.

Any of the tests described below may be used in addition to abdominal and rectal examinations to diagnose IBS. Most people with IBS appear to be healthy. So if the results are negative, don't worry; it simply means you have IBS and not anything more serious.

Occult blood test

The word occult means "hidden"—and this test is used to check for the presence of hidden blood in the stools. It is a routine way for screening for the early signs of bowel cancer. A small amount of stool is spread onto a paper which has been impregnated with one of several chemicals that react with blood by changing colour.

Cleaning your teeth too hard the night before can produce a positive result because it can make your gums bleed, and if you swallow blood then traces of it may be picked up by the test. Eating lightly cooked red meat, which contains blood, can produce a similar effect. Because of these possibilities for confusion, the test is normally repeated several times to confirm the result.

Stool culture

If you are suffering from recurrent diarrhoea or have had diarrhoea for a prolonged period, normally more than two weeks, this test will be carried out on a sample of

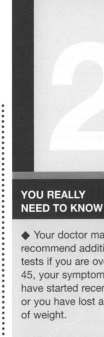

WHAT DOES IT MEAN?

OCCULT

Hidden; an occult blood test is carried out to detect blood hidden in the stools.

LACTOSE

A sugar present in milk. Some people do not produce lactase, the enzyme necessary to digest it, resulting in IBS-like symptoms, bloating, abdominal pain, flatulence and diarrhoea.

your stool to check for infections. Viral infections, bacteria such as *E. coli*, *Campylobacter*, salmonella and shigella, and parasites can all lead to diarrhoea. Bacterial infection is usually accompanied by vomiting, however.

Lactose tolerance testing

Because the symptoms of lactose intolerance are similar to those of IBS—diarrhoea, pain, bloating and wind—it may be necessary to rule out this condition.

There are several ways of testing for it. In the most commonly used method, you will be asked to drink a solution of lactose sugar. A blood sample will be taken, then further samples at 15, 30, 60, 90 and 120 minutes later, to check how well the lactose is being digested by the body. Any pain, flatulence, diarrhoea or bloating will also be checked for throughout the test. The blood is usually taken from a special line inserted into a vein in your wrist, so you won't have to have a needle inserted for each sample.

**YOU REALLY
NEED TO KNOW**

◆ Your doctor may recommend additional tests if you are over 45, your symptoms have started recently or you have lost a lot of weight.

◆ The tests are intended to rule out the possibility of a more serious condition.

◆ If you have IBS, the test results will be negative.

Examining the bowel

DOs AND DON'Ts

Do follow all instructions about what to eat and drink before a test, or the result may be inconclusive and the test may have to be carried out again.

Don't worry if you have to undergo these tests— they can be a bit uncomfortable, but they are not painful.

Sigmoidoscopy

The most commonly used internal examination of the bowel is a sigmoidoscopy. It allows the doctor to examine the inner walls of the lower part of the large intestine, known as the sigmoid colon. The instrument used is a sigmoidoscope, a long narrow viewing tube with a light at the tip.

The sigmoidoscope is gently inserted through your anus and rectum and into the bowel. It pumps air ahead of itself to spread the walls of the bowel apart as it moves along. The process is uncomfortable rather than painful. However, the air pumped into the bowel can sometimes trigger IBS-like symptoms of pain and bloating.

Colonoscopy

This procedure is similar to sigmoidoscopy but the instrument used is longer and more flexible, allowing the doctor to inspect higher up the large intestine. It is very commonly done where IBS is suspected. You will be

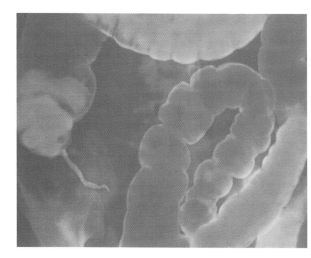

Coating the inside of the bowels with a solution of barium sulphate ensures that they will show up clearly on an x-ray image.

asked to take a laxative 10–14 hours before the investigation, to clean out the bowel, and will usually be given a sedative just before the procedure.

Barium enema

A routine method used in examinations for IBS, this test takes place in a hospital radiology department. The bowels do not show up on an x-ray, so an enema is given to coat the inside of the bowel with barium sulphate, a substance that the x-ray can pick up.

You will be asked to eat nothing the night before and to take a laxative to clean out the bowel. A small amount of barium solution will be pumped gently into your bowel via a tube inserted in your anus; x-rays are then taken.

Most of the barium solution will be expelled during your next bowel movement, but your stools may be chalky white for the next couple of days. It is important to expel the barium as quickly as possible as it can worsen constipation; taking a mild laxative can help.

Ultrasound

If gallstones are suspected, ultrasound will be used. It is a completely painless and non-invasive procedure in which a special probe is passed over the outside of your abdomen. The probe emits very high frequency sound waves which bounce back off the various internal organs. A computer analyses the returning sound waves and creates a picture of the internal organs on a screen.

Proctoscopy

Your doctor will carry out this test to detect haemorrhoids. A small instrument called a speculum is used to inspect the walls of the rectum for inflammation or bleeding.

YOU REALLY NEED TO KNOW

◆ It may be necessary to carry out a more thorough investigation of your bowel than the rectal examination done by your GP.

◆ These tests will be carried out in a hospital, not at your GP's surgery.

Examining the bowel

35

Aims of treatment

SELF HELP

Learn as much about your condition as you can, so that you can communicate with your doctor and work together to reduce your symptoms.

Be prepared to make lifestyle changes to keep your IBS under control.

IBS cannot be cured, nor do we know the cause in all but a minority of cases. Treatments for IBS therefore aim either to relieve the symptoms or to prevent them from recurring, or at least reduce their severity in the long term. Some treatments succeed in doing both. Eating more fibre, for example, may provide immediate relief from constipation; if the change to the diet is permanent, it may also prevent the constipation recurring.

Medical treatments

Drugs can certainly help alleviate diarrhoea and constipation, but they are only a short-term solution. All drugs have side effects, and some of these can, in the long run, make IBS symptoms worse. Nevertheless, a short course of drug therapy can give IBS sufferers a "breathing space" in which they can make changes to their diet and lifestyle to achieve a long-term improvement. For those concerned about the side effects of drugs, herbal medicine can offer a viable alternative (see p.54).

When IBS symptoms are severe, drugs to treat constipation or diarrhoea may be the best solution for short-term relief.

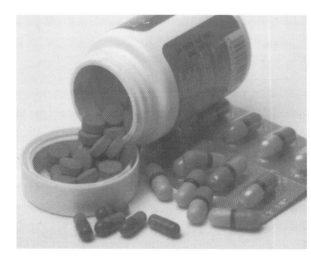

A CHRONIC CONDITION

Irritable bowel syndrome tends to be a long-term problem for many sufferers. It is what is known as a "chronic" condition. Examples of other chronic conditions are asthma and eczema. The term chronic condition is used to describe an illness or symptom that continues for a long period of time. The symptoms are intermittent and there may be occasions when there is very little evidence of them at all.

A flare-up of IBS may mean that instead of the odd bout of diarrhoea or constipation and the occasional spasm of pain, you suddenly begin to suffer severe symptoms, on a daily basis—severe enough to interfere with daily life. Some people with IBS lead perfectly normal lives most of the time, only to find themselves virtually housebound when the condition flares up.

Lifestyle changes

For many people, lifestyle changes are preferable to drugs for the long-term control of IBS symptoms.

Some people find that a change in diet is all that is needed to reduce or even banish their symptoms. As a general rule, a healthy balanced diet rich in fibre is best. If a food intolerance is exacerbating symptoms, it will be necessary to identify and eliminate the culprit food.

Therapies that help to reduce stress are often extremely beneficial in IBS. Counselling, psychotherapy, hypnotherapy and relaxation techniques such as yoga, meditation and aromatherapy can all be effective in reducing stress levels (see pp.56–63).

YOU REALLY NEED TO KNOW

◆ There are many drugs available that can treat the symptoms of IBS, but they may cause problems in the long term.

◆ Lifestyle changes such as improving diet or reducing stress levels may be the best option for long-term control of symptoms.

Aims of treatment

Treatment for constipation

There are four main types of laxatives: bulking agents; stool softeners; osmotic agents and stimulant laxatives.

TYPES OF LAXATIVES

TYPE	WHAT THEY ARE
BULKING AGENTS Natural bran Ispaghula Methylcellulose	Manufactured bulking agents are made from fibre and are taken as tablets or sprinkled over food.
STOOL SOFTENERS Docusate sodium	As the name suggests, this type of laxative softens the stools, allowing the bowel to push them along faster and making them easier to pass.

HOW THEY WORK

Bulking agents work by making the stools bulkier and softer. This allows the bowel to push them along faster and makes them easier to pass.

COMMENTS

Bulking agents work slowly and gently and are the safest form of laxative to take. It is very important to drink lots of water when taking them. You will need to be patient as they can take several days to work. They are usually taken in small amounts to begin with and the dose is gradually increased until a regular pattern of bowel movement is established. Bulking agents are safe to use over extended periods of time.

Stool softeners work in much the same way as detergents, breaking up the surface tension of the stool to allow it to absorb more water, making it softer.

Stool softeners take a day or two to work. They are given in quite large amounts at first and these doses are reduced once the laxative begins to work.

YOU REALLY NEED TO KNOW

◆ In the long run, it is better to include more fibre in your diet than to rely on bulking agents.

◆ Bulking agents are the most suitable constipation treatment for IBS sufferers.

◆ Prolonged use of laxatives can lead to bowel damage.

◆ Liquid paraffin is sometimes used as a stool softener, but this is not advisable—it can prevent vitamin absorption, lead to serious lung problems if inhaled and cause rectal irritation.

Treatment for constipation

There are several types of drugs available to treat constipation, all working in different ways, and some more suitable than others for IBS sufferers.

LAXATIVES

TYPE OF LAXATIVE	WHAT THEY ARE
OSMOTIC AGENTS Magnesium sulphate Magnesium hydroxide Sodium sulphate Sodium potassium tartrate	These are salts of sodium, magnesium or potassium and they normally work within three hours. They include many common over-the-counter remedies for constipation.
STIMULANT LAXATIVES Bisacodyl Senna	Stimulant laxatives use irritating substances. They generally take between six and 12 hours to work and can cause cramping abdominal pain.
ENEMAS Sodium salts	A fluid injected through the anus into the rectum; most enemas come in a tube or bag with a nozzle applicator.

HOW THEY WORK

Osmotic laxatives work by drawing large amounts of water into the large intestine to make the stools soft and loose. The water also triggers contractions which speed the passage of the stools through the intestine.

A laxative that irritates the walls of the large intestine, stimulating it to contract and propel the stools along.

The fluid softens and loosens any hard dry faeces stuck in the rectum.

COMMENTS

Drink lots of water when taking osmotic laxatives to avoid dehydration. Osmotics containing sodium should not be taken by people with high blood pressure or heart, liver or kidney problems. Osmotics containing magnesium should not be taken by people with kidney problems.

Repeated use can damage the bowel or leave it unable to function properly without the laxative. Stimulant laxatives are not generally recommended for people with IBS as they make other symptoms worse.

Many substances can be used, including olive oil and simple soapy water.

YOU REALLY NEED TO KNOW

◆ You should stop taking laxatives as soon as normal bowel function is restored.

◆ Stimulant laxatives may produce a bowel movement followed by a further bout of constipation.

◆ Laxatives are not a long-term solution for constipation caused by IBS.

Treatment for diarrhoea

DOs AND DON'Ts

✓ Drink plenty of water to replace the fluids lost during a bout of diarrhoea.

✗ Don't continue to take any anti-diarrhoeal drug long-term unless under medical supervision.

Many IBS sufferers will experience bouts of diarrhoea, especially first thing in the morning and after meals. Taking an over-the-counter anti-diarrhoeal drug can help control the problem but should only be regarded as a temporary measure. To avoid dehydration it is important to replace the fluids that are lost during a bout of diarrhoea. If your diarrhoea persists for more than a few days, consult a doctor.

Types of anti-diarrhoeal drug

The majority of drugs used to treat diarrhoea not caused by a bacterial infection fall into two categories according to how they work: those that act on the bowel wall and those that alter the contents of the bowel.

WHAT DOES IT MEAN?

BACTERIAL INFECTION
An infection by micro-organisms not normally present in the body. Diarrhoea is often caused by a bacterial infection in the bowel, but in IBS this is not the case.

OPIATE
A drug containing opium or a form of opium. Opiates have a sedative effect and cause drowsiness, and are addictive if taken regularly.

INERT
Something that does not react chemically. Inert substances are not metabolized by the body and pass harmlessly through the digestive system.

Drugs that act on the bowel wall

Opiate drugs are used to stop diarrhoea and reduce the painful spasms that accompany it, which they do by slowing down the contractions of the bowel wall. This group of drugs includes loperamide (the most common ingredient in over-the-counter medications for diarrhoea), co-phenotrope (a mixture of diphenoxylate and atropine) and codeine phosphate.

Codeine is converted by the body into morphine and, although the dose needed to stop diarrhoea is much smaller than that which produces side effects, nevertheless it should only be used occasionally. Long-term use of drugs containing codeine can cause the body to become more tolerant of it, so that more and more of the drug is needed to produce the same effect, which may eventually lead to dependence.

Drugs that alter bowel contents

There are two types of drugs that are used to relieve diarrhoea by altering the bowel contents: bulking agents and inert powders.

Bulking agents, which are mainly used to treat constipation (see p.38) can often make diarrhoea worse, but they do work for some people, so they may be worth a try. They work by absorbing excess fluid in the large intestine. This produces larger stools, which helps the bowel return to normality. However, they may take several days to work.

Inert powders mix with the excess fluid in the large intestine and help to carry away irritating or poisonous substances. Ingredients used include calcium carbonate (chalk), charcoal, aluminium salts (such as kaolin) and pectin (made from citrus fruits).

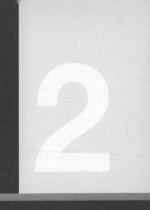

YOU REALLY NEED TO KNOW

◆ Always consult your doctor if diarrhoea lasts for more than a few days.

◆ Drugs to treat diarrhoea should be seen as a temporary measure and not taken over long periods of time.

◆ Long-term use of opiates can lead to dependence.

Treating other symptoms

Some of the other symptoms of IBS, such as abdominal pain, bloating and wind, may be sufficiently distressing to require treatment with drugs.

Antispasmodic drugs

As the name suggests, antispasmodic drugs prevent the sudden contractions of the bowel walls that cause colicky pain. They include dicyclomine and propantheline. However, many people with IBS find they are not helpful and that they cause unpleasant side effects including headaches, blurred vision, dry mouth, rashes, abdominal pain and constipation.

Antidepressants

Some people with IBS are helped by a drug known as a tricyclic antidepressant. If your doctor suggests this to you it does not necessarily mean that he or she thinks that your symptoms are the result of depression. Some people with IBS may indeed be depressed. However, whether their depression causes their symptoms or whether their symptoms contribute to their depression is a moot point.

The way in which tricyclic antidepressants work in IBS is not yet understood. They may work directly to reduce contractions and spasm in the walls of the bowel or, on the other hand, they may decrease the amount of pain that results from these events.

Tricyclic antidepressants can produce unpleasant side effects, especially in the first week or two of treatment. These can include a dry mouth, blurred vision and difficulty in passing urine. Unfortunately, tricyclic antidepressants can also cause constipation which makes them unsuitable for some people with IBS.

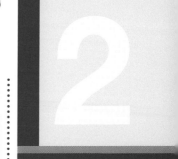

PEPPERMINT OIL

Peppermint oil contains menthol, which has an antispasmodic effect on the bowel walls, causing them to relax. Some gastroenterologists use it during colonoscopy (see p.34), squirting it directly on the mucous lining of the colon to relax it so the colonoscope can be inserted further without causing discomfort. Many people with IBS find it eases symptoms of pain, wind and particularly bloating. Peppermint oil is taken in the form of capsules which should be swallowed half an hour before meals.

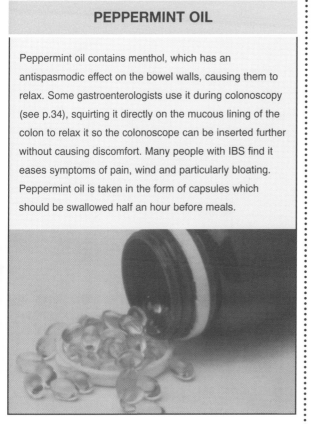

Self-help for bloating and wind

Try drinking peppermint, chamomile or fennel herb teas at regular intervals throughout the day. Alternatively, steep a sprig of fresh dill in a cup of boiling water for five minutes and drink the tea. Ginger can also help to reduce wind. Mix 5 ml (1 level teaspoon) into a cup of boiling water. Prepare and drink as often as desired. Ginger can also be taken as a tincture (see Herbal Medicine, pp.54–55); add about 10 drops to any herb tea and drink.

(see p.34)

YOU REALLY NEED TO KNOW

◆ If you are suffering from severe abdominal pain, antispasmodic drugs may help in the short term; ask your doctor.

◆ Antidepressants are sometimes prescribed for IBS because they relieve the physical symptoms—not because the patient is depressed.

Chapter

NON-MEDICAL APPROACHES

Getting more fibre

✓ Foods naturally rich in fibre are a better source than bran or supplements.

✗ Not all IBS sufferers benefit from a fibre-rich diet.

Although it doesn't work for all sufferers, many people with IBS find that including more fibre in their diet helps reduce their symptoms. A high-fibre diet may also slow the progress of diverticulosis and reduce the risk of cancer of the colon, so it is therefore a sensible approach for all people with or without IBS.

How to get more fibre

The best long-term way to obtain more fibre in your diet is to eat more fibre-rich foods: fruit, vegetables, and whole grains such as brown rice and bread are all good sources of natural fibre, but you can also boost your consumption by sprinkling bran over your food or by taking fibre supplements. It is important to drink plenty of water—several large glasses a day—at the same time.

Take it slowly

Don't overdo it, as this may make your symptoms worse and put you off before you feel any benefit. Make the change gradually to give your body time to adjust. If

HOW FIBRE HELPS

CONSTIPATION

Fibre provides bulk for the stools, making them solid but also soft. This helps the bowel move its contents smoothly and regularly.

DIARRHOEA

Additional fibre can absorb excessive fluid in the bowel and help to produce well-formed stools.

A FIBRE-RICH DIET

Getting more fibre needn't mean a radical change to your diet. Substitute fibre-rich versions for the refined foods you normally eat: wholemeal bread instead of white, and so on. The following are ideas on adding fibre to everyday meals:

TYPICAL MEAL	FIBRE-RICH VERSION
◆ Breakfast: Cornflakes, white toast with marmalade, tea or coffee.	◆ Breakfast: Bran cereal, wholemeal toast with marmalade, freshly squeezed orange juice, tea or coffee.
◆ Lunch: Cheese sandwich on white bread, cup of instant soup.	◆ Lunch: Cheese sandwich with tomato and lettuce on brown bread, piece of fruit.
◆ Dinner: Chicken with white rice, frozen peas, piece of chocolate cake.	◆ Dinner: Chicken with brown rice, frozen peas and roast parsnips, apple crumble made with wholegrain flour.

increasing your fibre intake does make some symptoms worse at first, try to stick with it. Most people find that these problems go away after two or three weeks and that, gradually, over the following months their bowel movements become regular and their other symptoms improve significantly, but it is important to be patient.

YOU REALLY NEED TO KNOW

◆ Increasing your fibre intake can be particularly helpful if the main problem is constipation.

◆ It is best to increase your fibre intake gradually, and allow plenty of time for any improvement in symptoms to appear.

Getting more fibre

Problem foods

If eating more fibre makes your symptoms worse and things do not improve within two or three weeks it may be because, like many people with IBS, you are unusually sensitive to certain foods.

A minority of IBS sufferers have a food intolerance—that is, their bodies are unable to cope with certain foods. Coeliac disease is an example of this. In most cases, however, IBS symptoms are not a result of food intolerance, but simply an exaggeration of the normal effects of food in the hypersensitive bowel. For example, caffeine stimulates the bowel in most people, but in an IBS sufferer it may cause diarrhoea and abdominal pain.

Cutting out foods

Eliminating a problem food may be all that is necessary to improve your symptoms, although in some cases this could mean far-reaching changes to your diet.

When cutting out foods, do so for only a few days. If your symptoms improve, leading you to believe that the food concerned is causing your symptoms, consult your doctor before making long-term changes to your diet.

Gluten intolerance

A minor percentage of people with a diagnosis of IBS are in fact suffering from coeliac disease (see p.22) and are unable to tolerate gluten, a protein in many cereals including wheat, oats, barley and rye. It may be worth cutting gluten out of your diet for a few days to see whether your symptoms improve. A gluten-free diet does not always produce a rapid improvement in symptoms, so the experiment may be inconclusive. If you still suspect that gluten is the problem, talk to your doctor, who may refer you for special antibody tests.

"Gassy" foods

If you are troubled by bloating and wind, try avoiding pulses, cabbage and other "gassy" foods. In a vegetarian diet, however, pulses are an important source of protein. One way to reduce their "gassy" effect is to soak them well—preferably overnight—before cooking.

Sorbitol

Many people with IBS find that the artificial sweetener sorbitol, often used in diabetic or low-calorie foods and in sugar-free chewing gum, triggers their symptoms.

Natural sugars

Fructose, a fruit sugar, is another common ingredient which some people find troublesome. Lactose, a sugar found in milk, can also cause IBS-type symptoms.

TOP TEN PROBLEM FOODS

A study of patients with food intolerances, carried out at Addenbrooke's Hospital in Cambridge, ranked problem foods according to the percentage of patients who suffered a reaction. The top ten foods were:

FOOD	%	FOOD	%
Wheat	60	Coffee	33
Corn	44	Rye	30
Milk	44	Eggs	26
Cheese	39	Tea	25
Oats	34	Citrus fruits	24

YOU REALLY NEED TO KNOW

◆ Some IBS sufferers experience a great improvement in symptoms when they cut out problem foods.

◆ Some of the most common problem foods play a major part in our diet. Wheat flour is used in most breads, biscuits, cakes, pasta and many breakfast cereals.

Elimination diets

A number of IBS sufferers find that certain foods or drinks trigger their symptoms. If this is the case for you, removing the offending substance may reduce the frequency of your symptoms.

Is food really the cause?

The link between IBS and food intolerance is controversial. Some sufferers undoubtedly have food intolerances; others are highly sensitive to foods that stimulate the bowel and will do well to avoid them. However, some studies have shown that secretly re-introducing foods into the diets of IBS sufferers after they have identified them as triggering symptoms does not cause a deterioration in their condition.

A sense of perspective

It is important to keep problem foods in perspective. The majority of IBS sufferers are not food intolerant, though they may well feel better if they don't eat foods that stimulate the bowel. It is not always necessary to eliminate a food completely—just reducing your intake may help. With milk, for example, some people find that they can tolerate a little in tea or coffee, when drinking a glass of milk would lead to an abrupt attack of diarrhoea. For some sufferers, just reviewing their diet in the light of healthy eating guidelines can help.

Identifying problem foods

Start by keeping a detailed food and drink diary for a couple of weeks. This may seem tedious, but the information it provides will be worth the effort. At the same time, keep a record of your symptoms—every bowel movement, the consistency of the stools, whether you had pain and, if so, how much (try rating pain on a scale of one to ten). Keep a record of your emotional state and menstrual cycle, too, to check whether your symptoms are affected by your mood. At the end of the fortnight you should have a good idea of which foodstuffs, if any, are producing symptoms.

Eliminating problem foods

Once you have identified the potential culprit, try cutting it out of your diet for a few days and then re-introducing it. Make a careful note of your symptoms before and after removing a particular food and after re-introducing it. This is known as a simple elimination or exclusion diet.

If you have identified more than one troublesome food, do not cut them out without professional advice, or you may be exchanging your IBS symptoms for nutritional deficiencies.

SEEKING PROFESSIONAL HELP

If you think that your symptoms are being caused by a number of foods, seek professional help before drastically reducing your diet. Your doctor can refer you to a dietician or nutritionist. You may have to go on a multiple exclusion or restriction diet, more complex versions of the simple exclusion diet in which several potentially troublesome foods are removed, and re-introduced one by one.

If you find that you have a food intolerance or are sensitive to several foods, your dietician will help you to find good alternatives so that you can still eat a balanced and healthy diet.

Herbal treatment

Do consult a herbalist —herbs contain powerful active ingredients and can have drastic effects.

Don't try to prepare your own herbal remedies from raw ingredients.

Herbal medicine can be extremely helpful to IBS sufferers. Some herbal remedies have direct beneficial effects on the digestive system and, if taken under the supervision of a qualified medical herbalist, they have few, if any, unwanted side effects. It is important in chronic conditions like IBS, in which symptoms may come and go for years, to have "safe" treatment at hand to deal with these as and when they arise.

Consult a professional

It is important to make a distinction between the treatment offered by a professional medical herbalist and over-the-counter herbal remedies. A herbalist will examine you and discuss your overall state of health, physical and emotional, as well as your IBS symptoms, before prescribing a remedy tailor-made for your needs.

Some people do find that pre-packaged herbal remedies help ease their IBS symptoms—everyone is different and it is worth trying some to find out. Generally, however, professional treatment is more effective.

A word of warning

Although herbal remedies are popularly regarded as gentle alternatives to conventional medicines, herbs are powerful substances and can be dangerous if misused. Taking a pre-packaged remedy will be safe enough if you follow the instructions, but never try to make your own remedies—always seek professional help.

Herbal preparations

The most familiar preparation is an infusion, or "tea"; the fresh or dried leaves or flowers of the plant are steeped in hot water for about 15 minutes, then the liquid is drained off and drunk. Decoctions (made by a similar method, but with hard parts of a plant, such as roots, seeds and bark) and tinctures (a mixture of water and alcohol in which herbs have been soaked) are more complicated to prepare, and are best obtained from a herbalist.

HERBAL REMEDIES FOR IBS

SYMPTOMS	REMEDY
PAINFUL SPASMS, BLOATING, WIND	Peppermint, chamomile or fennel, taken in infusion. Take any time. Avoid high doses of fennel in pregnancy.
PAINFUL SPASMS	Valerian: soak 1 level teaspoon powder in a tall glass of water overnight, or take tincture or tablets. Take any time. Wild yam: infusion of 1 teaspoon with 500 ml water, or take tincture or tablets. Avoid when pregnant.
DIARRHOEA, NAUSEA	Slippery elm: mix 1 level teaspoon powder in tall glass of water or take capsules. Take three times daily before meals.

Talking therapies

SELF-HELP

✓ Keep a record of your symptoms and emotional state to see if a pattern emerges.

✗ Do not talk to family or friends if it makes you uncomfortable— your doctor will be able to recommend a counsellor.

You may find that your symptoms are triggered or worsened by periods of stress and tension. This is not really surprising. Stress and anxiety can cause bowel symptoms in most people, and all the more so in IBS sufferers, where the bowel is hypersensitive.

IBS is associated with anxiety and sufferers continually score higher on scales designed to measure anxiety levels. It is also associated with depression and "illness attitudes" such as hypochondria and disease phobia. For some sufferers, therefore, counselling and psychotherapy can address these problems and help to reduce symptoms.

How do they work?

At their simplest, these therapies can help you find ways to tackle difficult problems and so reduce the stress that is contributing to your symptoms. Psychotherapy can

STRESS AND IBS SYMPTOMS

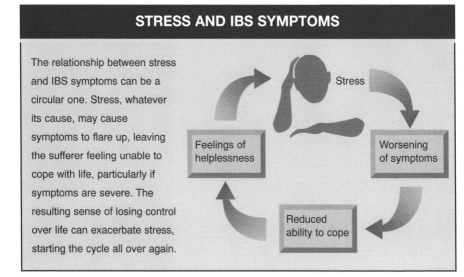

The relationship between stress and IBS symptoms can be a circular one. Stress, whatever its cause, may cause symptoms to flare up, leaving the sufferer feeling unable to cope with life, particularly if symptoms are severe. The resulting sense of losing control over life can exacerbate stress, starting the cycle all over again.

Stress

Worsening of symptoms

Reduced ability to cope

Feelings of helplessness

also help identify and resolve deeper areas of emotional conflict that manifest themselves in physical symptoms, although you may not be conscious of them day to day.

Counselling

A counsellor can provide a sympathetic and practical listening ear in a safe environment, allowing you to talk about and sort out your problems.

We have all experienced the relief of talking over a particularly worrying problem with a good friend. Talking through a problem is the first step towards dealing with it or, if that is not possible, accepting it and moving on.

Sometimes we can deal with problems by discussing them with family and friends. However, it is not always easy to discuss personal problems—marital difficulties, for example—with a close family member or friend without involving them in distress and worry. It can be better to have a listener who is not as emotionally close as our family and friends and can give objective advice. This is what a counsellor does.

Psychotherapy

As with counsellors, psychotherapists talk with their patients. This form of counselling explores the individual's deep-seated, and often subconscious, conflicts and emotions, examining their effect on his or her everyday life. Psychotherapists may work with the people who consult them by using methods such as role play, helping to identify and understand their underlying problems and find ways of solving them.

Psychotherapy is not the same as psychiatry. Unlike psychiatrists, psychotherapists are not usually medically trained doctors and do not prescribe drugs.

YOU REALLY NEED TO KNOW

◆ Counsellors lend a sympathetic, objective and practical listening ear to help sort out problems.

◆ Psychotherapy helps identify and resolve subconscious conflicts which can produce physical symptoms.

Talking therapies

Hypnotherapy

FACTS

Hypnotherapy has been approved as a useful medical tool by the American Medical Association since 1958.

You cannot be made to act against your will while in a hypnotic trance.

Hypnotherapy, the healing of a person while they are in a trance-like state, or hypnotized, is one of the most effective treatments for IBS. Many sufferers find their symptoms improve greatly after only a short course of treatment and that the improvement lasts.

Hypnotherapy is one of the best-researched and most widely used complementary therapies. It is used at hospitals and research centres around the world to treat a wide range of health problems. As well as IBS, hypnotherapy can treat chronic pain, migraine, many stress-related conditions, anxiety, depression, phobias and addiction, and can reduce pain during childbirth.

How hypnotherapy works

Scientists have been trying to discover for many years exactly how hypnotherapy works. It is now thought that hypnosis puts the two sides of the brain—the left which tends to deal with language and logic, and the right which handles emotions and symbolism—in closer communication with each other. This allows connections between behaviour and its underlying causes to be identified and understood. Whether or not this is true,

A WORD OF WARNING

Like most medical techniques, hypnosis is very safe in skilled hands. However, it is a powerful tool and can be dangerous if mishandled. For this reason it is important to consult a properly qualified practitioner, preferably a medical doctor or dentist or, failing that, someone with training in clinical psychology.

VISUALIZATION

A hypnotherapist may induce your trance by inviting you to imagine a place where you feel comfortable, a room at home, a tropical beach or a forest glade. Think of a scene where you feel safe and able to relax.

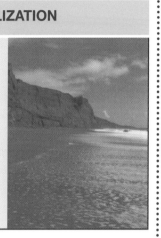

hypnotherapy is essentially a relaxation therapy. During a hypnotic trance the body relaxes deeply in much the same way as during meditation. The heart rate slows, breathing deepens and blood pressure decreases. While in the trance, you are more open to suggestion, and this is the key to dealing with problems through hypnosis.

Hypnotherapy in practice

The practitioner will talk to you for a while and then ask you to imagine you are drifting or sinking into comfort. As you relax, your eyelids will begin to feel heavy and your eyes will close. You will then be in a light hypnotic trance. You will feel you are between waking and sleeping, aware of everything around you but detached from it. You can speak and end the trance whenever you wish.

Once you are in a trance, the practitioner can look for subconscious causes of your symptoms. When these have been found, he or she can suggest solutions to you, aiming to replace negative thought patterns with positive ones.

Hypnotherapy

Meditation

Research shows that daily meditation can improve both mental and physical health; many IBS sufferers find that regular meditation brings about a marked improvement in their symptoms or, in some cases, can even eliminate them altogether.

In addition to IBS it has been shown to help with high blood pressure, chronic pain, asthma and heart disease. During meditation the heart rate and breathing rate both decrease and brain activity alters to patterns only seen during very deep relaxation. Those who meditate regularly have described feelings of well-being, mental clarity and peace.

The scientific basis

Scientific investigation into the effects of meditation was pioneered in the 1960s by the American researcher Dr Herbert Benson. He came up with the term "relaxation

LEARNING TO MEDITATE

◆ Choose a warm, comfortable room, quiet and not too bright. Take the phone off the hook. Sit comfortably on a chair or on the floor, making sure your back is straight.

◆ You may find it helps to concentrate on an object such as a candle flame, visualize a pleasant scene, or close your eyes and repeat a word or phrase in your head.

◆ Do not try to concentrate your mind; try to allow it to become empty.

◆ If your mind wanders, accept this and do not become irritated by it; just gently return your concentration to your meditation object. With practice, you will do this almost without thought.

◆ Be patient with yourself; meditation takes practice.

◆ Breathe slowly and regularly, through the nose rather than the mouth and into the abdomen rather than the chest (see p.74).

BENEFITS OF MEDITATION

Practised regularly, meditation can help you control some of the triggers that aggravate the symptoms of IBS, such as stress and tension by:

◆ Lowering the heart rate.

◆ Reducing blood pressure.

◆ Relaxing the muscles.

◆ Helping to alleviate insomnia.

response" to describe the physical effects of meditation and noted that these were the direct opposite of the body's adrenaline-induced "fight or flight" response— the instinctive human reaction to stress, fear and danger —when the heart and breathing rate both increase.

Transcendental meditation

Often referred to as simply TM, Transcendental meditation is the most popular form of meditation in the developed Western world. Most of the research into the health benefits of meditation has involved TM.

Practitioners of TM repeat short words or phrases (known as mantras) in their heads to help them over-come conscious thought and reach what is called a state of "deep consciousness" or "thought-free awareness". This stage transcends thought (hence the name) and allows the individual direct access to their energy and creative "centre".

YOU REALLY NEED TO KNOW

◆ Meditation is a form of relaxation therapy.

◆ Regular meditation (15 to 20 minutes twice a day) can improve IBS symptoms or prevent them returning.

◆ Meditation takes practice and it may be best to join a class to learn the technique.

Meditation

Aromatherapy and yoga

DOs AND DON'Ts

✓ Do attend a yoga class at first so you can learn the postures properly.

✗ Some aromatherapy oils should not be used by those with high blood pressure, kidney disease or during pregnancy. Check with an aromatherapist first.

Many other complementary therapies can be helpful in reducing stress, but two of the most useful for sufferers from IBS are aromatherapy and yoga.

Aromatherapy

Aromatherapy uses essential plant oils to produce therapeutic effects. The oils are extracted from the flower, buds or root of the plant, or from the fruit peel (citrus oils). Extraction methods include distillation and expression (squeezing or pressing).

Each oil has its own characteristic aroma. Some oils have specific medicinal properties; lavender, for example, is antiseptic. Others have an effect on mood; some are soothing, others are stimulating. Massaging the abdomen with essential oils is relaxing and can help to ease the symptoms of IBS.

USING ESSENTIAL OILS

Essential oils are extremely strong and are used in tiny amounts. They should be added to a much larger amount of a "carrier" oil such as wheatgerm, sweet almond or grapeseed before they are used.

To prepare oils for an aromatherapy massage, add between two and five drops of essential oil to 10 ml of carrier oil and shake well. The proportion of essential oil in the blend should not exceed 3 percent, whether you are using a single essential oil or a combination.

For an abdominal massage to soothe IBS symptoms try a mixture of essential oils of peppermint and black pepper or, alternatively, rosemary and marjoram.

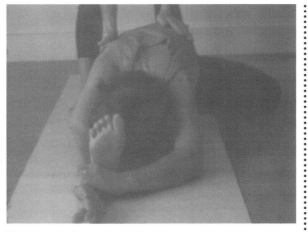

Yoga is a good overall relaxation therapy, and certain positions are reputed to aid digestion and bowel function.

Yoga

The health benefits of yoga have been researched for many years. Regular practice has been shown to reduce high blood pressure, lower levels of anxiety and stress and promote relaxation.

An ancient Indian system of breathing and body exercises, yoga is actually a complete philosophy in itself which aims, eventually, to bring the individual into harmony with the universe. However, the vast majority of Westerners who practise yoga do so simply because it helps keep them fit and supple and promotes a sense of well-being and relaxation.

You can teach yourself yoga from a book but it is always better to attend a class, at least to begin with, as it is important to learn the various postures properly. For maximum benefits, it is recommended that you practise yoga on a regular basis—ideally every day—rather than just attending a class once a week.

YOU REALLY NEED TO KNOW

◆ Massaging the abdomen with essential oils can ease IBS symptoms.

◆ Essential oils should be used with a much larger amount of "carrier" oil.

◆ Regular yoga practice reduces blood pressure, relieves anxiety and stress and promotes relaxation.

Aromatherapy and yoga

Chapter

LIVING WITH IBS

Improving your diet

✓ Overcooking fruit and vegetables can destroy the nutrients they contain.

✗ Avoid tea and coffee as they are diuretics, drink herbal tea or water instead if you want to boost your fluid intake.

Even if your IBS symptoms are not caused by a food intolerance, improving your diet may prevent them from flaring up. As a general principle, avoid processed foods and "ready meals", which generally contain additives, and aim for a wholefood diet packed with fresh foods.

Whole grains

The importance of fibre to normal bowel function is well established. Choose whole-grain versions of foods rather than their refined counterparts to add fibre to your diet.

Fruit and vegetables

Eaten raw, or lightly cooked for maximum nutritional value, fruit and vegetables are excellant sources of fibre and contain essential vitamins and minerals. Eat fresh fruit between meals rather than fatty or sugary foods.

Water

Drink plenty of water. This is especially important if you are constipated, though you should also drink lots of water during bouts of diarrhoea to avoid dehydration.

The human body needs at least 1.5 litres (2½ pints) of water a day—the amount shown here—to stay healthy. Drink water with meals, and sip water or herbal tea throughout the day to get your quota.

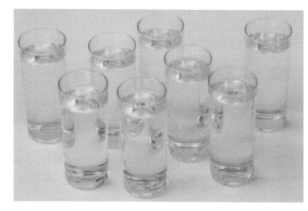

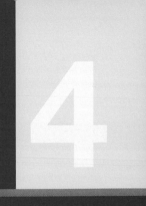

HOW TO EAT

In a condition such as IBS, in which both diet and stress can play important roles, how you eat can be just as important as what you eat.

◆ Have small meals at regular times throughout the day—this is easier for the digestive system to handle than a lot of snacking and one big meal.

◆ Always make time for breakfast, however busy you are—if necessary, get up 15 minutes earlier in the morning.

◆ Eat a substantial lunch.

◆ Make your evening meal the lightest of the day, and eat at 7 or 8pm rather than 10pm to give your body time to begin digesting your food before bedtime.

◆ Never rush a meal or eat "on the run". Make time to eat in a leisurely fashion.

◆ Sit down to eat, concentrate on what you are eating and chew food thoroughly.

Yoghurt

The balance of micro-organisms in the bowel can be upset by a bout of gastroenteritis ("holiday tummy"), triggering IBS symptoms. To help the bowel replenish the levels of healthy bacteria, try eating plenty of natural, unsweetened "live" yoghurt.

The beneficial ingredient in "live" yoghurt is a bacterium called *Lactobacillus acidophilus*; you can take this in the form of a daily supplement if you prefer.

YOU REALLY NEED TO KNOW

◆ Eat a wholefood diet with plenty of fruit and vegetables—aim for five servings a day.

◆ Drink at least 1.5 litres (2½ pints) of water a day.

◆ Eat your main meal around midday, not in the evening.

Improving your diet

Foods to avoid

DOs AND DON'Ts

✓ If you cut out a food, try to replace it with one that contains similar nutrients.

✗ Don't try to change your diet radically over night; it will be difficult to stick to the new diet, and you may even worsen your symptoms.

Some of the foods discussed here are best avoided or eaten only in limited quantities by anyone who wants to have a healthy diet. Others are mentioned because they can trigger symptoms in some IBS sufferers—you may have to experiment to see whether this is true for you.

In addition to the foods listed here, some people have intolerances (see p.48) to "windy" foods such as beans, lentils, brussels sprouts, peas and cabbage, the artificial sweetener sorbitol, used extensively in so-called "diet" products and in sugar-free chewing gum, and the fruit sugar fructose.

Red meat

Many people with IBS find that eating red meat triggers their symptoms, so it may be worth cutting it out to see whether this helps. Eat fish and poultry instead to make sure you are getting enough protein, and whole grains and dark green vegetables to maintain your supply of iron.

Saturated fats

Most of us eat too much fat, and saturated fat—the kind present in foods of animal origin, such as meat and dairy produce—can be harmful to health. Reduce your intake by switching from full-fat to semi-skimmed or skimmed milk, and replacing cream with low-fat fromage frais. Spread butter thinly on your bread (do not replace it with margarine, which is a highly refined product containing preservatives and additives). Eat only small amounts of cheese; about 40g (1½ ounces) daily is enough.

Foods that are fried or roasted absorb large amounts of fat so try to keep these methods of cooking to an absolute minimum. As a general rule you should steam, grill, casserole or bake food instead.

Spicy foods

Many people with IBS find that foods which are heavily spiced—some Indian dishes for example—make their symptoms worse. Note your symptoms after your next meal containing spicy food to see if this applies to you.

Caffeine

Because caffeine can have a powerful effect on bowel function, it is worth cutting out tea, coffee and colas, to see whether this helps. You will not lose out nutritionally by doing this, as long as your overall fluid intake remains sufficient. Switch to water and herbal teas instead.

Alcohol

In some people alcohol can irritate the bowel, especially if drunk in excess. A couple of glasses of wine a day is unlikely to make much difference. However, it may be worth cutting out alcohol completely for a while to see if you are particularly sensitive to its effects. If you do drink alcohol, always accompany it with some food.

**YOU REALLY
NEED TO KNOW**

◆ The information on food packaging usually includes the saturated fat content of the food, so you can check it.

◆ Caffeine is present not only in tea and coffee, but also in chocolate and cola drinks.

MODERATE YOUR DIET

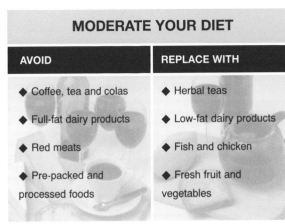

AVOID	REPLACE WITH
◆ Coffee, tea and colas	◆ Herbal teas
◆ Full-fat dairy products	◆ Low-fat dairy products
◆ Red meats	◆ Fish and chicken
◆ Pre-packed and processed foods	◆ Fresh fruit and vegetables

Foods to avoid

Dealing with stress

✓ Make a list of the things that cause you to become stressed and decide which you can change and which you can't.

✗ Don't try to do it all alone; think of practical solutions for the things you can change, and enlist any support you need for those you can't.

In many cases there is a clear relationship between IBS symptoms and stress. Taking action to reduce your stress levels is therefore an important step towards improving your symptoms.

Why is stress bad?

Not all stress is bad. Happy events, such as getting married or being promoted at work, can cause stress but because we view these things in a positive way, we generally take the uncertainty they cause in our stride.

Stress is an inevitable part of being alive. A life wholly without stress, where everything was predictable and no effort was ever required to deal with problems, would be a life without achievement or reward. Constant stress, however, can be harmful to health, particularly if you feel that you have no control over your situation.

Our reaction to different types of stress is highly individual. The important thing is to identify the situations which you personally find stressful, change them if you can and learn to live with them if you cannot. In order to cope better with unavoidable stresses it is often necessary to learn to relax (see pp.72–75) and view them in a positive rather than a negative way.

Plan to avoid stress

Each of us face routine situations every day which "wind us up". Avoidance can be the best method for removing these everyday stresses.

Reschedule your day. For example, if your journey to work is difficult and you are often late, allow more time. Leave home earlier to avoid the worst of the rush hour. It will mean getting up a bit earlier but that is a small price to pay for keeping your stress levels down.

Plan ahead. If shopping in a crowded supermarket makes your blood boil, try to do your shopping at less busy times. If you seem to end up queuing for ages every time you visit the post office, find out when the quiet periods are and go then whenever possible.

Unavoidable stress

Other sources of long-term stress, such as problems with family members, neighbours and work colleagues, may be less easy to deal with and ultimately you may have to learn to live with them. In this sort of complicated situation many people find that counselling (see p.54) can help them to understand their problems better and find, if not solutions, then ways of living with them.

MONEY WORRIES

Money is one of life's biggest stressors. A realistic view of what you need and what you can afford combined with a bit of forward planning can go a long way towards reducing the stress.

Try to budget your expenditure. Allow for bills that will be coming along in the next few months and put aside the money to pay them before they become due. If you have run up a large credit card bill, plan to pay it off in regular instalments—work out what you can afford each month and how long it will take to pay the total.

Taking control of your finances in this way may seem complicated and time-consuming at first, but after the initial effort it will become much easier, and it will relieve you of a great deal of worry.

YOU REALLY NEED TO KNOW

◆ Stress plays a major role in IBS.

◆ Taking positive action to deal with problems will increase your sense of control over events and help reduce stress.

◆ Setting aside some time each day just for yourself can prevent stress from building up over time.

A less stressful lifestyle

✓ Make time for stress-reduction activities. Schedule them in your diary and treat them with the same importance that you would treat an appointment.

✗ Don't ignore the signs that you are becoming stressed— such as irritability or sleeplessness.

Whatever the specific stresses in your life, they will be easier to deal with if you are physically fit, rested and have a positive self-image. Some basic lifestyle changes can go a long way towards reducing your stress levels. In addition to the advice given here, good diet and eating habits (see pp.64–5) are also an important part of a stress-reducing lifestyle.

Exercise
Regular aerobic exercise can improve IBS symptoms, help you relax and sleep better, get you fit, build a better self-image and encourage positive thinking. Aim to exercise for 20 minutes at least three times a week. Choose a form of exercise that leaves you slightly breathless, such as jogging, swimming or cycling.

Get enough sleep
Most people need seven to eight hours' sleep a night. Get into the habit of going to bed and getting up at a regular time. Reserve your bedroom for sleeping and lovemaking—don't watch TV, eat or work there. Avoid eating and drinking late at night as this can prevent you from sleeping properly. Ensure your bed is comfortable.

Cut out smoking
If you smoke, try to give up or at least cut down. Nicotine has a powerful effect on bowel function and quitting will help reduce your symptoms.

Drink in moderation
Many people feel that having a few drinks helps them to relax, but in the long run, the opposite is the case, particularly with excessive drinking. Too much alcohol can

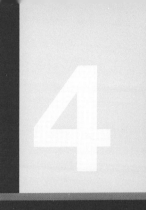

irritate the bowel. Don't drink on an empty stomach. At a party or similar function, pace your drinking by alternating alcoholic drinks with glasses of water.

Relaxation

Try to put some time aside each day, even if it is only 30 minutes or so, to relax. This should be your time, a space in the day when you unwind and forget about the family, the bills, work and all your other worries.

During this period, switch off the TV and take the phone off the hook—or turn down the volume on the answering machine—and do something that relaxes you. Have a candlelit bath, diffuse an aromatic essential oil in your bedroom and simply lie down and drift away, read a book or take the dog for a walk—whatever works for you.

EXERCISE

Taking regular exercise can be very beneficial in relieving the symptoms of IBS: it helps to reduce stress levels, and also the discomfort of bloating and distension.

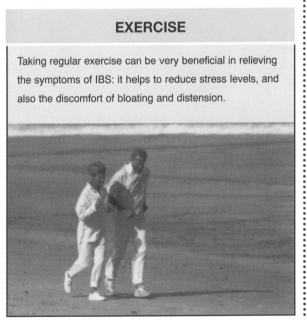

A less stressful lifestyle

Breathing and relaxation

SELF HELP

Learn to observe your chest and abdomen so you can tell whether you are breathing correctly.

Practise the breathing exercise so that you can switch to relaxed breathing at will.

Breathing correctly is an important aid to handling stress. There are two ways of breathing and the body employs them in different situations.

Relaxed breathing

When your breathing is relaxed, the diaphragm—the dome-shaped muscle that separates the chest from the abdomen—contracts, pushing the contents of the abdomen down and creating a vacuum in the chest which causes air to be sucked into the lungs. The diaphragm then relaxes and the contents of the abdomen rise back up, forcing air back out of the lungs.

TENSE BREATHING

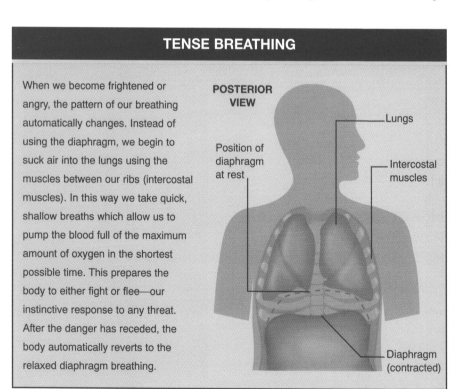

When we become frightened or angry, the pattern of our breathing automatically changes. Instead of using the diaphragm, we begin to suck air into the lungs using the muscles between our ribs (intercostal muscles). In this way we take quick, shallow breaths which allow us to pump the blood full of the maximum amount of oxygen in the shortest possible time. This prepares the body to either fight or flee—our instinctive response to any threat. After the danger has receded, the body automatically reverts to the relaxed diaphragm breathing.

POSTERIOR VIEW

Position of diaphragm at rest

Lungs

Intercostal muscles

Diaphragm (contracted)

A SIMPLE BREATHING EXERCISE

Lie down in a quiet room. Close your eyes. Place one hand on your chest and the other on your abdomen just below the rib cage. Breathe in slowly, allowing your abdomen to push up. Breathe out and feel your abdomen flatten. This is breathing with the diaphragm—your chest should hardly move.

Breathe like this for several minutes, getting into an easy, slow rhythm, and you will feel yourself relax. When you are feeling stressed and upset, check your breathing. If you are breathing using your chest, gently correct the pattern by breathing into your abdomen.

With a bit of practice you will be able to do this anywhere—in your car in a traffic jam, at your desk, or in a supermarket queue.

YOU REALLY NEED TO KNOW

◆ Breathing correctly helps to reduce your stress levels.

◆ Normal, relaxed breathing uses the diaphragm, not the chest muscles.

When you breathe in this way, breathing in pushes out the front of your abdomen and breathing out allows it to flatten again.

How stress affects our breathing

During periods of long-term stress and anxiety it is often possible to get into the habit of tense incorrect breathing. This means that the body continues to run on "red alert", setting up a vicious circle of stress and tension which will eventually cause a variety of stress-induced health problems.

By becoming more aware of changes in your breathing pattern, you will be able to help yourself to relax by deliberately breathing with the diaphragm.

Breathing and relaxation

Understanding the jargon

Medicine is full of technical terms and words that can make a condition such as irritable bowel syndrome seem more daunting than it really is. Knowing what the terms mean can clarify your condition and enable you to communicate more easily with your doctor.

ALLERGY—a physical reaction which results when the body's immune system attacks a foreign substance. Asthma and eczema are common conditions involving allergic reactions.

ANAL FISSURE—a tear in the lining of the anal canal usually caused by passing very large, hard stools.

BARIUM ENEMA—a preparation of barium sulphate used to coat the inner bowel walls allowing them to be examined on x-ray. It is introduced into the bowel via a tube inserted in the anus.

COELIAC DISEASE—a condition in which the body cannot tolerate gluten, a protein found in cereals such as wheat, barley, rye and oats.

COLONOSCOPY—internal examination of the large intestine using a long flexible viewing tube with a light at the tip (colonoscope).

CONSTIPATION—usually defined as having a bowel motion less than twice a week or straining to pass stools more than 25 percent of the time.

DIARRHOEA—a loose consistency of stool with increased frequency of bowel motions.

DUODENUM—the upper part of the small intestine.

ENZYMES—chemicals produced by the digestive system to break down potentially toxic substances found in food and render them harmless.

FIBRE—the part of our food that we cannot digest. It passes through the digestive system and makes the stools bulkier, speeding their passage through the digestive system and making them easier to pass.

FLATULENCE (WIND)—the expulsion through the anus of waste gases from the digestive system.

FUNCTIONAL DISORDER—a change in the way a bodily process works (digestion in IBS), not caused by disease.

GASTROENTERITIS (HOLIDAY TUMMY)—nausea, vomiting and diarrhoea caused by a bacterial infection.

GASTROENTEROLOGY—the medical science concerned with problems of the digestive system.

HAEMORRHOIDS (PILES)—soft lumps which can develop in and around the anus as a result of straining to pass stools due to constipation.

ILEUM—the lowest part of the small intestine.

JEJUNUM—the middle section of the small intestine.

OESOPHAGUS—the tube leading from the throat to the stomach.

SYNDROME—a collection of symptoms which occur together and are associated with a single disorder.

ULTRASOUND—a non-invasive procedure which uses high-frequency sound waves to examine internal organs.

Understanding the jargon

Useful addresses

WHERE TO GO FOR HELP

**BRITISH DIGESTIVE
FOUNDATION**
3 St Andrews Place
London NW1 4LB
Tel: 020 7486 0341

**BRITISH HERBAL
MEDICINE ASSOCIATION**
Sun House
Church Street
Stroud GL5 1JL
Tel: 01453 751389

**BRITISH SOCIETY OF
MEDICAL AND DENTAL
HYPNOTHERAPISTS**
17 Keppel View Road
Kimberworth
Rotherham
South Yorks S61 2AR
Tel: 01709 554558

COELIAC SOCIETY
PO Box 220
High Wycombe
Bucks HP11 2HY
Tel: 01494 437278

**COUNCIL FOR
COMPLEMENTARY AND
ALTERNATIVE MEDICINE**
63 Jeddo Road
London W12 9ED
Tel: 020 8735 0632

IBS RESEARCH TEAM
Central Middlesex Hospital
NHS Trust
Helpline: 0336 411286
(calls cost 39p a minute off
peak, 49p a minute at
all other times)

IBS NETWORK
Northern General Hospital
Sheffield S5 7AU
www.ibsnetwork.org.uk

**WOMEN'S NUTRITIONAL
ADVISORY SERVICE**
PO Box 268
Lewes
East Sussex BN7 1QN
Tel: 01273 487366

Index

Index

Acknowledgements
SPL= Science Photo Library
Photographs: 19 Astrid & Hanns-Frieder Michler/SPL; 26 BSIP Chassenet/SPL;
28/29 Tek Image/SPL; 34 CNRI/SPL; 46/47 John Greim/SPL; 58/59 Sinclair Stammers/SPL;
63 Francoise Sauze/SPL; 64/65 BSIP, LECA/SPL; 73 Gable, Jerrican/SPL

Illustrations: Axis Design Editions Limited

This book was edited and designed by Axis Design Editions Limited,
8 Accommodation Road, London NW11 8ED